The 5:2 Diet:

The Beginner's Guide to Weight Loss Using the Fast Diet

I0429460

Table Of Contents

Introduction

I want to thank you and congratulate you for downloading *The 5:2 Diet: The Beginner's Guide to Weight Loss Using the Fast Diet*. There are literally thousands of weight loss plans and diets out there. Everyone seems to have their two cents when it comes to deciding which plan is right for you. From doctors and gurus, to a blogger online and your mother, information is being thrown at you from all sides and you honestly don't know what is best for you and your body. Well, look no further. The 5:2 Diet is the simplest dieting method that allows you to eat *whatever* you want and help you *lose weight*!

Starting by breaking down the basic science behind the 5:2 Diet, this book will provide you with everything you need to know about the 5:2 Diet; including how to implement it in your life. This book contains proven steps and strategies on how to lose weight and live a healthier life. Here is an inescapable fact: nothing is ever going to change if you don't at the very least start gathering some information about losing weight. You don't need to look any further than this book for everything you need to lose weight; whether it's twenty or seventy pounds.

Losing weight is all about self-development; it takes more than just a physical effort to make any progress. Working towards becoming a healthier and better you will take all the willpower you have combined with physical effort. But if you persist and persevere, there is no reason why you can't lose weight and live out your dreams.

It's time for you to become an amazing expert of the 5:2 Diet! Losing weight doesn't have to be a dreaded struggle. With these tips and recipes, you will be more ready than you ever have been before to accomplish your fitness goals and be the very best version of yourself. Good luck on your weight loss journey! Remember to never give up and always believe in yourself! Enjoy!

Chapter 1: What is the 5:2 Diet?

The 5:2 Diet is more than just a "fad diet." It is a lifestyle that allows people who want to lose weight and create a positive lifestyle achieve their goals without sacrificing their favorite foods. While most diets are given a set lifespan, say one to three months, the 5:2 Diet is structure for long-term sustainability with the outcome of legitimate results. You can still enjoy all of the delicious food you love and crave without torturing yourself with guilt or self-loathing. Often times, dieting means constricting your caloric intake and saying goodbye to your favorite snacks or desserts. However, your weight loss journey does not have to be defined by the amount of torture you put yourself through. A common struggle with many dieters is the feeling of guilt after losing control during a binge. But self-deprecation should not go hand-in-hand with dieting. This is why the 5:2 Diet is one of the most popular methods of losing weight. You don't have to worry about overeating or that a piece of bread has 120 calories. It is a simple alteration of your lifestyle that will feel normal after just a few weeks.

To put it simply, the 5:2 Diet is when you eat as you normally would for five days of the week. Then, on the other two days you greatly restrict the amount of calories you eat, these are called 'fasting days.' Fasting is normally associated with extreme exaggerations of starving oneself for days. But this is not how the 5:2 Diet works. You can still eat during your fast days, you are simply eating much less food than on your normal days. But before we go into the specifics and science behind the 5:2 Diet, you need to understand the greatest benefit and genius behind implementing intermittent fasting.

Intermittent Fasting

Intermittent fasting is when you fast for a pre-determined number of hours before eating. It is restricting your eating time so you don't over eat or snack. This method is especially beneficial for night owls or people who like to snack before going to bed. A typical intermittent fast is sixteen hours, beginning at 8 o'clock at night and ending at 12 noon the following day. During those sixteen hours you limit your food intake to just water and/or tea and coffee without sugar or cream added. While many 'experts' advise snacking or eating every four hours, the reality is that your body does not need a continuous stream of food to function. In fact, snacking and eating often prevents your body from burning all of the carbs and protein for fuel, leading to extra stored fat; which is the exact opposite of what you want.

Intermittent fasting should be structured to fit your schedule; the 8pm to noon structure is fitting for a standard 9 to 5 job. If you work the late shift or start working at 5am, then you need to figure out the best time that a sixteen hour intermittent fast works to your advantage. This is one of the greatest benefits of intermittent fasting; it works to make dieting and losing weight easier. Starting your fast at 8pm means that most of the time fasting is done when you are sleeping; so you are not thinking about food and worrying about getting cravings. By the time you wake up, you only have a few hours to go until you can enjoy a light meal.

But intermittent fasting is not just a great weight loss method; there are dozens of proven benefits that have been life changing for thousands of people. It helps your body repair its cells to prevent serious diseases, like heart disease, Alzheimer's, cancer, stroke, and type 2 diabetes. Many people have also shown improved blood pressure and cholesterol.

- Insulin levels drop drastically, increasing fat burning and weight loss success, as well as reversing some cases of diabetes.

- Growth hormone increases in your blood levels to facilitate muscle gain and fat burning.

- As your body begins cell repair, it removes toxic waste from your cells; resulting in better overall health.

- There are positive changes to your molecules and genes that promote a longer lifespan and protection against disease.

- Intermittent fasting reduces and prevents inflammation to promote overall health.

- Intermittent fasting has been shown to reduce the risk of cancer and ultimately cure it. Cancer is characterized by uncontrolled growth of cells. Fasting has given evidence of affecting the metabolism in a way that reduces the risk of cancer, as well as reducing some of the side effects of chemotherapy. Although there are not enough human studies to give enough voice to these findings, many people have shared their success stories with intermittent fasting and clean eating to help fight their cancer.

With all of these amazing and miraculous benefits associated with intermittent fasting, it is hard to believe that it is not a widely accepted method of weight loss or healthy living. However, there are many vocal individuals who share their experiences with intermittent fasting online and in books in an attempt to spread the word about this incredible lifestyle.

Fasting Days

Now that you understand intermittent fasting a bit better, you can learn more about what happens on a fasting day during the 5:2 diet. On your two fast days you restrict your calorie consumption to only 25% of your caloric needs. The purpose of restricting your caloric intake is to insinuate weight loss and make you more aware of what you eat. Becoming more aware of what you eat leads you to making healthier choices and really savoring every meal you eat. Choosing a healthier alternative to a hot Italian sub for lunch can lead to increased energy and less sugar cravings.

You never have to go without food on your fast days, you just have to eat a quarter of the calories you normally would. The average female would be reduced to a 500 calorie diet, and the average male would be restricted to 600 calories. The limitation allows you to consume three small meals a day. Some people even work their way to doing a complete fast, consuming absolutely no food or sugary drinks on their fasting days. There are online calculators that will help you determine your exact calorie intake for your normal days and your fasting days.

Theoretically you can eat what you want on a fast day, as long as you stay within the calorie limit. However, to last the day on a restricted diet, eating the right foods will make you feel full without wasting calories. There are two fasting days in the 5:2 Diet. But that does not mean that you have to fast for two consecutive days. Many people who first start the diet decide to not fast for two days in a row, and split up the fasts with a few days in between. Splitting up the days makes the hunger pangs and cravings easier to manage. However, back-to-back fasts may be more convenient and produce results faster. It is important to not exceed 48 hours of fasting if you do choose to do a complete two day fast.

Normal Days

The standard caloric maintenance intake for women is around 2,000 calories, while men are recommended to intake around 2,400 calories each day. The exact number of calories that you should intake can be determined by calculators online. Your personal calorie intake is unique to the individual, based on your body mass index, basal metabolic rate, and total daily energy expenditure.

Your Body Mass Index or BMI is a calculation of your body fat percentage based on your weight, weights, and sometimes age. Although a BMI chart or scale can be found online and in your doctor's office, it is not always an accurate assessment of your health. The standard charts are not accurate for pregnant women, individuals with muscular builds, young children, and individuals under five feet tall.

Your Basal Metabolic Rate or BMR is the amount of calories you burn during twenty-four hours of not being active. It can be difficult to determine your BMR, but there are calculators online to help you find your basal metabolic rate.

Your Total Daily Energy Expenditure or TDEE is the amount of calories you burn in a day scaling your basal metabolic rate level of activity. Your TDEE is the amount of calories you need to burn on a daily basis to maintain your present weight. It is the number of calories you should consume on your normal days. Your total daily energy expenditure is dependent on how active you are; the more calories you burn exercising, the better.

Many people tend to overestimate how much exercise they actually do. When you are calculating your TDEE and are doubtful of your activity level, just choose a lower activity level. Here is a detailed explanation of each activity level, so you know where you fall on the activity scale.

Activity Level

Sedentary- This is when you incorporate little to no exercise each day. Sedentary is the level for people who do not or cannot include exercise as part of their daily routine.

Lightly Active- This is when you incorporate light exercise or sports 1 to 3 days a week. This level includes individuals who walk everyday but do not have an actual workout regime.

Moderately Active- This is when you incorporate a decent amount of exercise or sports 3 to 5 days a week. This level is for individuals who are active for at least thirty minutes at a time daily, at least three times a week.

Very Active- This is when you are exercise or play sports at a significant level or intensity 6 to 7 days a week. This level includes serious but non-professional athletes who consistently train for a goal that requires daily hard exercise, lasting for at least an hour each day.

Extremely Active- This is when you do very hard exercise or sports more than once a day, in addition to a physical job. This level is for people who have multiple workouts each day for at least one hour at a time. Their job typically entails them to maintain top physical form. This is not a common level, most active athletes in training will identify with "very active" most of the time.

Chapter 2: How to Implement the 5:2 Diet

Just like any major lifestyle adjustment, the 5:2 Diet takes an action plan and real change to produce legitimate results. Even when you are eating within your calorie limit, eating the wrong food can inhibit or stop your progress, resulting in a weight loss plateau or even weight gain. This does not necessarily mean that you should only eat salads or skip dessert. The key to success is implementing a strict but practical diet plan that will guarantee results while keeping you full with a happy tummy.

Provided in this chapter is a detailed grocery shopping list. But before we dive right into what you should and shouldn't eat, let's go over why the food choices described are important for your weight loss diet.

- Eating large portions of vegetables will keep you full, while providing good carbs, vitamins, and other nutrients your body needs. Especially leafy green vegetables like lettuce, spinach, and kale.

- Opting for smaller meat portions will give you the right amount of protein while limiting your unhealthy fats intake. You should bake, grill, or roast your meat, rather than fry it. Meat also tends to make you feel full even when consuming it in smaller portions.

- Making soups a regular part of your diet is a great way to add in vegetables and other yummy food while keeping your calorie count low. Many major soup brands offer heart healthy low calorie choices for individuals who are on a diet.

- Eggs are a breakfast staple. They offer protein and good fats to give you energy for a long day head.

- Cutting out processed carbohydrates will do wonders for your weight loss journey. Bread, rice, pasta, and other grain products along with sugary foods keep your body from burning fat and can lead to weight gain and plateaus. If you start craving something sweet, it is best to opt for berries or other low sugar fruits to curb your cravings.

- Drinking plenty of water, tea, and black coffee will help heal and detox your digestive system to help your body process the food you eat. Although you should stay away from food and beverages with "sugar free" labels, due to artificial sweeteners. Artificial sweeteners are actually worse for your body than natural sugar. They have a long list of side effects, including: headaches, migraines, weigh gain, cancer, memory loss, dizziness, depression, joint pain, slurred speech, blurred vision, muscle spasms, and cramps. You should also remember that what you drink counts as your caloric intake, so don't forget to record them when you are adding up your calories at the end of the day.

You 5:2 Diet Shopping List

Eating smart starts with a prepared grocery list that sets up your meals for at least the next week. The food you buy at the beginning of the week should be prepped for the following six days. Prepping your meals keeps you from spontaneous bingeing or unplanned calories that could ruin your diet for the day. You do not have to worry or think about what you are going to eat for dinner because it is already made at home. The grocery list provided is not to limit your food choices, but to give you a good sense of the right foods to buy so you can make even more progress. You can eat whatever you want when on the 5:2 diet, this list is just an outline of a good, healthy diet.

Here is a sample of an ideal grocery list for the 5:2 Diet:

- Vegetables

    - Green Beans
    - Broccoli
    - Cauliflower

- Spinach
- Kale
- Lettuce
- Celery
- Beets
- Radishes
- Onions
- Peppers
- Peas
- Beans
- Carrots
- Sweet Potatoes
- Hummus

- Fruits
  - Apples
  - Cherries
  - Blueberries
  - Grapes
  - Pears
  - Melon
  - Bananas
  - Blackberries
  - Raspberries
  - Strawberries
- Meat
  - Chicken
  - Pork
  - Beef
  - Seafood/ Fish
  - Lamb
  - Turkey
  - Eggs
- Grains
  - Whole Wheat/Grain Bread
  - Tortillas
  - Whole Wheat Pasta
  - Brown Rice
  - Oatmeal
- Cheese
- Nuts

- Nut Butter
- Organic Dark Chocolate
- Yogurt

Chapter 3: Curbing Your Cravings

Cravings can be the biggest struggle when trying to lose weight. One minute you are doing great and are proud for sticking with the meal plan for so long, then the next minute you're trying to stop yourself from indulging in a brownie sundae. Temptation is going to hit you hard, so it is important to know how to fight off a bingeing session and avoid losing control. Many circumstance may arise that will require you to improvise with your diet. Whether it's a work party or going out to eat with some friends, you do not want to be caught off guard and make a rash decision that can ruin your calorie count for the day. Here are ten great tips that will help your curb any cravings and keep your goals on track!

1. Get enough sleep! Sleeping helps your body rebuild cells, repair damage, and reboot so you can function the next day. Getting too little or too much sleep can cause you to make bad decisions that could hurt your progress. Loss of sleep will increase your appetite, leading to massive cravings. Make sure you are getting between six to eight hours of sleep every night for weight loss success.

2. Start the day right by eating a healthy breakfast! Some people on the 5:2 Diet prefer to skip breakfast all together, especially during or after a fasting day. This is completely fine, but the first meal you do eat should be enough to fill you up and give you enough energy to work. Work in a breakfast that is high in protein and fiber to control sugar cravings. Most people tend to eat a high carb breakfast, resulting in short bursts of energy followed by sudden drops and fatigue. Sticking to scrambled eggs and a packet of oatmeal will fill your tummy while keeping your energy up.

3. Fight your hunger! Many people eat without actually feeling hungry. Eating every four to six hours will not give you a chance to experience true hunger. Sometimes when you give in to your hunger, you end up eating a lot more than

you initially planned. Eating whole grains and vegetables will keep you from giving into hunger and help you fight sugar cravings.

4. Stick to a schedule. Don't just pre –make your meals, set specific times for when you should eat them. Manage your hunger by only eating at set time and avoiding snacking.

5. Plan for cravings. Curbing your cravings does not necessarily mean that sugary foods are off limits. You should plan to crave something sweet and add in a small 100 calorie treat to your meals.

6. Don't keep temptation in your house! The worst thing you can do is keep yummy sugary foods in the house or at work. You should make the foods you crave difficult to get to. Cravings do pass, so subjecting yourself to knowing that a delicious brownie is taunting you in the fridge will only make stay strong more challenging.

7. Find an alternative to your unhealthy food trigger. There are more than a dozen different healthy alternatives to the typical sweets that you normally enjoy. Eating fruit, yogurt, dark chocolate, or nuts will keep you from splurging on an unhealthy processed snack. Find an alternative that has fewer calories and more fiber and protein to fill you up while curbing your sweet tooth.

8. Write it down! Keep a food diary or journal to record your cravings. This can keep you from giving in to temptation and help fight your cravings in the future. Writing down when and what you are craving will help you identify the time of day when your temptation is the strongest, making it easier to plan an alternative snack ahead of time.

9. Note your triggers. Emotional and stress eating are real struggles for many people. If you can identify your craving triggers, you can understand and control what you eat and how you react.

10. There is a stigma about diets that you have to eat the same boring and bland foods every day. Even though

limiting what you eat can help you manage your calories, it can make eating seem like a chore. Keep a varied diet to keep your taste buds excited. Just because you are on a diet does not mean that you can't be satisfied and enjoy your meals.

Chapter 4: The Most Common Mistakes of the 5:2 Diet

1. When you hear "eat whatever you like," you actually hear "eat however much you like." On normal eating days you can eat whatever you want: cake, ice cream, tacos, whatever. But eating whatever you like does not mean that you can eat as much of it as you want, especially when you are trying to lose weight. The idea of the 5:2 diet is to reduce your calorie consumption over as the week goes and learning to focus on what you are eating and how it affects your body. Consistently eating over your calorie budget will negate the caloric deficit of your fasting days and will inhibit any weight loss.

2. Counting your calories incorrectly. This is one of the biggest mistakes people make on the 5:2 Diet. First be sure that you are consuming the right amount of calories. Regardless of which online calculator you use to determine how many you should intake, the numbers should be accurate. Secondly, make sure that you are taking a minute to read the nutrition label on your food. There shouldn't be any second guessing with what you eat because most foods have an accurate calorie count on the label. Also, be sure to take into account the number of servings you are consuming. A standard nutrition label only shows what is in one serving of the product you are consuming, even when there may be more than one serving in the container or package. Always re-read the nutrition label and keep track of your servings. Of course, fresh fruits and vegetables are much harder to keep track of because they do not come with nutrition labels. You can easily find the estimated nutritional value of fresh foods online.

3. Not giving yourself enough credit when needed. "Failing" is subject, in a way. And not giving yourself the benefit of the

doubt can cause you to unnecessarily rethink your diet plans and goals. If you go over your calorie count on a fast day, do not punish yourself or feel guilty. Going a few calories over on your fast day is not going to hurt your fast. Going significantly over your calorie count can slightly impact your weight loss, but not enough to make you feel bad about eat a bit over budget. Intermittent fasting is a lifestyle that takes time to get used to; and you are going to have many fasting days ahead of you. So do not beat yourself up just because one of them went slightly south. Just learn from your mistakes and see your next fast day as another chance to do better.

4. Eating back the calories you burn is another mistake that can hurt your weight loss. Exercising is a great way to lose weight, burn calories, and feel great. You should definitely add in some exercise days into your week to help you reach your goals faster. However, even if you burn a significant amount of calories at the gym, you should not eat it all back at dinner. The calories you burn from exercising are not added into your calorie allowance for the day. Consider the calories you burn exercising as a bonus.

5. Breaking your fast too soon is another common mistake. Your fasting days are twenty-four hours long, just like any other day. Going to sleep at 6pm and waking up at 11pm to have a late night snack still counts towards your fasting day allowance. Wait until the next day to begin eating normally again. In reality, fasting days are actually longer than twenty-four hours because you get a full night's sleep again before eating normally. So staying up until midnight on your fasting day so you can eat something does not count as an added meal to your normal day. Not to mention that staying up late to eat after a fasting day is bad for your sleeping habits and can inhibit weight loss.

6. Indulging during the last meal before your fasting day is a mistake that can hurt your fast. Consuming too much food before a fast will make it harder for your body to detox during the fast. Instead of eating anything you can get your

hands on during your last normal meal, you should eat something smaller and healthier.

7. Going into a fast blind is one of the worst methods of handling a fast. You should have a meal plan ready to go before you begin your fasting day, so you will not be tempted to eat more than your calorie allowance.

8. Sharing your fasting days with the world is not part of the 5:2 Diet. Regardless of whether you are looking forward to your fast day or dreading it, there is no need to tell everyone you know. Bringing in outsiders to look on as spectators to your dieting experience may cause unnecessary social pressure. What if you actually did badly on your fasting day? What if your friends and family voice doubt instead of support? If you really want to share your fasting experience and talk about it, then make sure you are sharing it with someone who is only going to offer support and encouragement.

9. Indulging right after a fast is one of the worst things you can do on the 5:2 diet. Fasting is to cleanse your body and help you lose weight. Eating a trunk load of junk after a successful fast will defeat the purpose of the fast. All of your hard work will have been for nothing. Your body is not meant to handle extreme eating habits. So, after you fast, try breaking it with a small, light, and healthy meal.

Chapter 5: 3 Month Meal Plan for Success

Some people find it difficult to come up with a strategic meal plan that will fit their dietary needs, as well as their work schedule. The meal plan listed below is just a few examples of high protein and fiber meals that will keep you on track and feel full to help you achieve as much success as possible!

Breakfast

1. A medium bowl of oatmeal with a tablespoon of blanched almonds. Served with one sliced apple.

2. Two scrambled eggs with cheese, served with one slice of whole grain toast and half an apple.

3. Crumbled feta cheese with half an avocado with lime juice on whole grain toast.

4. Half a cup of full fat Greek yogurt with half a cup of mixed berries.

5. Two sliced of roasted ham with two poached eggs and a slice of cheese.

6. One two-egg omelet with a handful of wilted spinach. Served with one slice of whole grain toast.

7. Breakfast smoothie- one banana mixed with Greek yogurt and one teaspoon of vanilla extract. Pour in half a cup of milk to thin it out.

8. Two poached eggs on wilted spinach, served with one sliced apple.

9. One scrambled egg with one small chopped tomato, served with a handful of spinach and a diced mushroom.

10. Make a fruit medley with one cut up banana, two sliced kiwis, and a half a cup of blueberries.

Lunch

1. Poached salmon with a mixed salad, topped with olive oil and lemon juice.

2. Chicken Caesar salad topped with chickpeas, served with olive oil on top.

3. Chicken and veggie soup served with four rye crackers.

4. Mushroom soup served with one apple.

5. Roasted vegetable cous cous served with delicious carrot sticks.

6. Potato salad made with capers, mustard, and gherkins.

7. Grilled chicken wrap made with a whole wheat tortilla, tomatoes, low sodium cheese, and lettuce.

8. Spinach salad tossed with parmesan cheese, apple slices, and one boiled egg sliced up.

9. Mixed bean salad served with mustard and carrot sticks.

10. Cooked chicken served with steamed broccoli, topped with low sodium soy sauce.

Dinner

1. 6 0z. fillet steak served with one baked sweet potato and steamed green beans.

2. Grilled sea bass served with roasted vegetable stir fry.

3. Grilled or baked salmon served with a spinach side salad.

4. One large Portobello mushroom, stuffed with lentils and four artichoke hearts. Drizzle a little olive oil on top for some extra flavor.

5. Chili served with sour cream and cedar cheese.

6. Beef stew served over brown rice with a side of your favorite vegetable.

7. Pork tenderloins served with sauerkraut and cauliflower.

8. Veggie spaghetti served with olive oil, with a side of cooked carrots and peas.

9. Roasted cod served with brown rice and broccoli.

10. Stuffed peppers served with a mixed leaf side salad.

Snacks and Desserts

1. ¼ of an organic dark chocolate bar.

2. ½ cup of almonds.

3. 2 tablespoons of nut butter.

4. 1 cup of vanilla ice cream or frozen yogurt.

5. Fruit and cottage cheese.

6. Natural lightly buttered popcorn.

7. Yogurt parfait.

8. One graham cracker with peanut butter.

9. One baked apple served with nuts.

10. Trail mix with chocolate.

Conclusion

Thank you again for downloading this book!

I hope this book was able to help you to understand the 5:2 Diet, as well as motivate you to work for your goals and maybe even set new ones!

The next step is to use everything you learned in this book, from detoxing to a new dinner idea, and apply it in your everyday life! Creating a new lifestyle takes time, effort, motivation, and excitement! Using the information that you read is the only way any positive change is going to come your way. So take action and start becoming a better and healthier you!

Finally, if you enjoyed this book, please take the time to share your thoughts and post a review on Amazon. It'd be greatly appreciated!

Thank you and good luck!

Crossfit Diet

The complete guide to getting started with the Crossfit diet

Introduction

I want to thank you and congratulate you for downloading the book, *"Crossfit Diet: The complete guide to getting started with the crossfit diet"*.

This book contains proven steps and strategies on how to get started with the crossfit diet that can effectively provide your body with the right sustenance it needs while you do the workouts. Crossfit training can help you lose weight, enhance your strength and stamina, provides balance, and make you feel good about yourself.

The crossfit workouts are more rigid than your usual exercises, and you will see positive results if you do it on regular basis. To effectively pull it off, you need to eat the right diet that will be able to support your body while training. This book can help you decide for the right foods to eat and succeed in your endeavor.

You also need to have patience, discipline, diligence, and will power to help yourself see the results that you want to see.

Thanks again for downloading this book, I hope you enjoy it!

Chapter 1: Crossfit Diet 101: Understanding What Crossfit is and the Diet that Works

Crossfit is a complete fitness program. Its creator Greg Glassman, a former gymnast, involved a combination of several workouts to come up with the most effective set of exercises for an athlete. The exercises include cardiovascular workouts, functional strength training, and intense athletic movements. The crossfitter needs to give his body the right sustenance it needs to cope up with the rigid exercises that the program requires to give the maximum benefit.

Among the available diet programs around, the Paleo diet works well (and it is the most suitable diet) with the set of exercises that the crossfit program requires. The Paleo diet follows a dietary guideline based on the presumed early diet of the Paleolithic men. This diet requires nuts, vegetables, fruit, fish, and meat (pork, chicken, or beef). It is taboo to include dairy, legumes, grain, and processed food in a Paleo diet – to sum it up, do not eat any kind of food that did not exist during the Paleolithic age.

Every type of food in a Paleo diet is exactly the kind of food that a crossfitter needs to consume. It will give him the right sustenance that can help him with his crossfit training. The Paleo diet can provide the right amount of protein, fiber, and other necessary nutrients that he will need as he trains. But still, you need to modify the Paleo diet in order to fit into your crossfitter life.

Your deeper understanding regarding the foods that you are allowed and not allowed to eat in a Paleo diet can help you plan your meal – something that you and your whole family could share. Your family will surely love the succulent dishes that they won't mind eating the dishes that you prepared while following the protocols in the Paleo diet program. You will learn more about Paleo Diet in Chapter 2, and some of the succulent dishes in Chapter 4.

Advantages of Crossfit Diet Over the other Diet Programs

The required crossfit diet of the crosfitter is the same as the Paleo diet. There should be a lot of protein and other important nutrients. You also need to consume lots of water to replenish the lost liquid during the training or workout.

The Paleo diet is the most ideal diet program to follow when doing crossfit training. You don't need to closely monitor the calories of each food you take, as long as you have the right proportion of food on your plate. You also need to keep in mind the kinds of food that the early men usually eat during the Paleolithic period.

You won't be deprived of flavors when you switch to Paleo diet. There are a lot of recipes that offer succulent dishes that are tailored for Paleo diet. You can serve the same dish to your entire family and get them fit in no time.

There are guilt-free desserts that you can try. Paleo diet uses natural sweeteners to whip up a tasty dessert. You are not permitted to use processed sugar granules, aside from the fact that sugar can bring more harm to your body than good. Some uses Stevia, honey, or molasses when creating their own dessert recipe. Never use artificial sweeteners because they are packed with preservatives that can only harm your body.

When you switch to Paleo diet, you won't feel like you are following a diet program. You can cook anything within the specified list of food that you can eat, and you practically don't need to measure each portion to take. It is easy and simple to follow, and you won't starve.

If you do crossfit training, you need a well fed body to avoid breaking down. The other diet programs tend to make you hungry because you need to burn more calories if you do crossfit workout. If you limit your caloric intake, then there's a huge possibility that your body won't be able to cope. The ideal crossfit diet, the Paleo diet, won't make your body starve and you can work out for long hours. You might need to slightly modify the Paleo diet to fit into your training.

The Crossfit Nutrition

Crossfit has its own dietary guidelines that the crossfitter needs to follow together with the exercises in the crossfit training.

The official CrossFit website says that the needed nutrients should follow this proportion: 40% carbohydrates, 30 % protein, and 30% fat. A crossfitter can get the needed amount of nutrients by eating only vegetables, nuts, lean meats, and seeds. The CrossFit website further states that the diets that are high in carbohydrates have the power to raise a person's insulin levels. An increased insulin level can lead to obesity and occurrence of chronic disease. You can find the complete list of good sources of carbohydrates, protein, and fat on Chapter 2.

The CrossFit organization also believes that a reduced calorie has the ability to promote longevity. It also decreases the risks of having heart disease and/or cancer.

You need to learn to eat only quality foods that your body needs. For most people, this is something hard to do. Those who are used to having bread, grains, and other processed carbohydrates are likely to give up if they can't part with the said foods. But, if you are someone who is determined to succeed in your endeavor, then you need to learn how to control yourself from consuming the taboo foods that the crossfit diet strictly prohibits. You need to shop for lean meats, fruits and vegetables, nuts, and seeds. It is not recommended to switch abruptly to crossfit diet, you can try small changes in your diet each day until you get used to it. Small, regular, and sustained changes are the things that you need to keep in mind when switching to the crossfit diet.

You are Already Eating Quality Foods

If you are accustomed to eating quality foods, the next thing you need to learn is how to get the right proportions of your quality foods that will give you the amount of fuel that you need for your workout. Supplying your body with the right quantity of fuel will prevent breakdown.

It is recommended that you consume the suggested proportions in "The Crossfit Nutrition" section of this book. It is also recommended that you take regular small meals throughout the day.

What about my Family?

To be blunt, you will never hear any complaints from your family about the meal if you can give them something succulent yet won't defy your diet program. Preparing two sets of meal (one for you, and one for the entire family) can invite an argument. Your family might feel alienated when you do that, and they might feel like you are separating yourself from them. It might even create barriers, which you don't want to happen.

If you can suggest recipes that you all can agree on (of course they are Paleo friendly recipes), then the problem will be solved in a matter of time. You need to include your family with certain decisions before you proceed with your plan. There are great recipes in this book that you will all surely agree on.

The earlier you start your kids with Paleo diet, the better. You can be certain that they will grow up healthy and fit, and they will carry that to their adult years. You don't need to worry too much about their health even if they have to part from you and leave home.

When Eating Out

Eating out with family and friends is something inevitable. You don't need to worry about sacrificing your diet or having fun – you can have fun while eating the required proportion in your crossfit diet. You can estimate the quality portion of your protein by using the palm of your hand – your meat should be about that big. You can choose your carbs from the list of fruits and vegetables found on Chapter 2. If you have a palm-sized steak, then you can have broccoli along with your steak.

Drinking Alcohol

Drinking alcohol is not prohibited, and a crosfitter is allowed to drink occasionally. Anything taken excessively, not just alcohol, is bad. There are crossfit athletes who consume alcohol once in a while and there are those who completely abstain from drinking alcohol. Most crossfit atheletes who gain success in their endeavor do not drink alcohol at all. To be frank, if you want to succeed, then it is best to stay away from alcohol.

Aside from the right diet and workout, you need to make sure that your body gets proper rest and you must sleep when it is time to sleep.

Chapter 2: Getting Started with the Crossfit Diet

Earlier, you learned that Paleo is the most ideal diet to follow if you are a crossfitter. This book assumes that you follow a regular regimen for your workout, and you need a suitable diet to meet your goal.

Paleo diet is the closest diet program that can sustain you body with all the needed nutrients and sustenance that it needs to satisfy the demands of the crossfit training. This book can help you modify your Paleo diet to perfectly fit into your crossfitter life. You need to gain a clear understanding regarding the foods that you can eat and not to eat on the Paleo diet. It can help a lot when you plan for your meal. Keep in mind that simplicity is beauty, and it only means that simpler meals are always better than complicated ones.

Your Food Guide

To make Paleo works for you it is important to think like a predator and don't act like a prey. What does that mean? Paleolithic men were meat eaters. You need to effectively mimic that time period, but we will modify it a bit. You are expected to eat organic meats as your protein source, good amount of fats, and some fruits and vegetables for your carbohydrates.

It is advisable to find grass-fed meat in the market if you can. Red meats like venison, bison (the meat source that closely resembles the one in the Paleolithic Age), goat, elk, and beef are the best choices. You can be certain that a grass-fed meat doesn't contain chemicals as compared to meats that were fed with feeds that contain different chemicals. Pork and chicken must be consumed in moderation, the excessive omega-6 they contain make them far less healthy.

It would be easier for you to plan your meal if you have a list of quality sources for your carbohydrates, fats, and protein.

Your Quality Carbohydrates

When you talk about quality carbohydrates you need to think about antioxidants. High quality carbs should be able to provide antioxidants and keeps the insulin and blood sugar levels as steady as possible.

The good sources of quality carbs are as follows:

Class	Food Items
Excellent Source of Carbohydrates	Vegetables:
	Cauliflower
	Broccoli
	Kale
	Romaine lettuce
	Spinach
	Fruits:
	Blackberries
	Blueberries
	Strawberries
Very Good Source of Carbohydrates	Vegetables:
	Cabbage
	Brussels sprouts
	Eggplant
	Onion
	Red pepper
	String beans
	Fruits:
	Kiwi

		Pink Grapefruit
		Plum
		Tomato
Good Source of Carbohydrates	Vegetables:	
		Celery
		Cucumber
		Yellow squash
	Fruits:	
		Green grapes
		Orange
		Pear
		Red grapes

Your Quality Protein

When you define the quality of a protein of a certain food source, you need to think about its fat content. Understand that all protein food sources, including tofu, have fat.

The good sources of quality protein are as follows:

Class	Food Items
Excellent Source of Protein	Cod
	Haddock
	Lobster
	Mackerel
	Salmon
	Sea bass
	Snapper
	Soybean hamburger crumbles

	Tuna steak
	Turkey breast
	Turkey breast, deli
Very Good Source of Protein	Chicken breast
	Chicken breast, deli
	Cottage cheese (1%)
	Emu
	Freshwater bass
	Trout
	Tuna, canned in water
	Soy imitation meat products
Good Source of Protein	Beef tenderloin, well-trimmed
	Pork tenderloin, well-trimmed
	Tempeh
	Tofu, extra-firm
	Tofu, firm
	Tofu, soft
Low-Quality Source of Protein	Bacon
	Ground beef (27% fat)
	Sausage

Your Quality Fats

You need quality fat to provide better fuel for your body. The best sources of quality fat are the foods that contain high concentration of monounsaturated fats and low in Omega-6 and saturated fats. The saturated fats can raise your cholesterol levels, which usually give heart disease.

The good sources of quality fats are as follows:

Class	Food Items
Excellent Source of Fats	Olives
	Olive oil
	Macadamia nuts
Very Good Quality Source of Fats	Almond butter
	Almonds
	Avocado
	Canola oil
Good Quality Source of Fats	Cashews
	Peanuts
Poor Quality Source of Fats	Butter
	Lard
	Soybean oil
	Safflower oil

If you can come up with a meal plan that includes the best sources of quality barbs, protein, and fats, then choose to do that. However, there are times when your body craves for the food sources that provide lesser benefits (but still considered an okay source of the needed nutrients); you can include them as well just make sure not to do it regularly. You won't be able to get used to eating quality foods if you always include foods that give lesser benefits. Yes, you should not include the foods that won't give any benefit at all.

Also, you need to completely stay away from junk foods, they bring nothing but trouble. It is recommended not to try them anymore, especially if you are already used to eating the recommended food sources.

Chapter 3: Your Very Own Paleo Staples

Preparing a Paleo meal in a jiffy is not always possible, and having a simple Paleo meal might become boring at one point. You might still crave for a more flavorful or fancier dish once in a while. Unfortunately, to make a flavorful dish you need to follow a recipe that is a bit complicated. The good news is you can still whip up a succulent meal within fifteen minutes if you have your basic and/or pre-cooked ingredients ready beforehand.

You can buy the Paleo staples in groceries or supermarkets, but you can't really be sure if you are buying something that is free from chemical preservatives and other ingredients that are not Paleo friendly. The only way to make sure is if you make the staples yourself.

Bone Broth

You can store this homemade bone broth in the freezer. It is recommended to use silicone muffin mold when freezing your broth. Let the broth cool first after making it. When it has cooled, get your silicon mold and carefully pour the broth in each muffin hole. Put the mold in the freezer and wait for it to turn solid. Remove the frozen broth from the mold and store it in Ziploc. The frozen broth is good within seven days.

You can prepare a quick soup using the frozen broth. You simply pop two or more broth blocks in a casserole, and heat the broth over low fire. Bring it to boil, and add some vegetables and pre-cooked meat to make a delightful quick soup.

Use a 6-quart pressure cooker to cook your broth.

Ingredients:

2 leaks, trimmed and halved
2 carrots, peeled and quartered
2.5 pounds of bones (choice of chicken, pork, or beef)
8 cups water
1 teaspoon apple cider vinegar
2 tablespoons salt

Procedure:

1. Put all the ingredients in the pressure cooker, lock it, and set it to high pressure.

2. Cook your ingredients over high heat.

3. Immediately bring down the cooker's temperature once it reached high pressure. Cook for thirty or more minutes.

4. Turn off the stove, and wait for the pressure inside the cooker to naturally release.

5. Strain the broth, and let it cool for a bit.

You can use a slow cooker if you don't have a pressure cooker, but expect it to take longer to cook.

Paleo Mayonnaise

It is good to use Paleo mayonnaise for dishes in your crossfit diet that need mayo. There is a lot of Paleo mayonnaise in the market, but you wouldn't know if the Paleo mayonnaise that you are buying is the real deal. To be safe, make your own Paleo mayonnaise, it's easy.

Ingredients:

2 yolks of organic eggs
Half teaspoon of salt
A pinch of white pepper
1 tablespoon Dijon mustard
2 tablespoons lemon juice
1½ cups macadamia or avocado oil

Procedure:

Use room temperature ingredients.

1. Combine all the ingredients in a steel or ceramic bowl, except oil.

2.   Beat or whip the ingredients until you get a smooth consistency.

3. Add the oil while whisking, make sure to add in thin stream.

4. If the mixture begins to cling to the sides of the bowl, then you can slowly stir in the remaining oil while you continue whisking.

You can store your fresh mayonnaise in the refrigerator to maximum of three days. You can drizzle some of it on your favorite greens after making it, and enjoy a truly guilt-free salad.

These Paleo staples are great help in preparing your Paleo dishes.

Chapter 4: Some Crossfit Recipes to Try

This chapter is dedicated to some of the ideal recipes you can try to start your crossfit diet. You can create different combinations of the dishes as you make a meal plan. There are different healthy dressings that you can try when you are on the go.

Caesar Dressing ala Paleo

The Caesar dressing is versatile enough to add in any salad, and you can use it as dip. You can add other spices to your liking or use it as it is.

Ingredients:

1 tablespoon lemon juice
2 tablespoons Paleo mayo
Half cup of olive oil, extra-virgin
5 cloves of garlic, minced
1 tablespoon Dijon mustard
Anchovy fillets, minced
Some ground black pepper and sea salt to taste

Procedure:

Use your blender to combine garlic, lemon juice, and mustard. Add the mayonnaise and continue blending. Slowly put in the olive oil while the blender keeps on going. After blending, use your spatula to scrape all the finished dressing in a bowl. Season it with salt and pepper; add a bit more of lemon juice together with the anchovy fillet. Taste and adjust.

Vinaigrette: Raspberry-Walnut

This vinaigrette is inspired by lemon vinaigrette. Instead of using lemon juice and olive oil, we will use raspberry vinegar and walnut oil.

Ingredients:

3 tablespoons raspberry vinegar
Half teaspoon of Dijon mustard

3/4 cup walnut oil
Salt and ground black pepper to taste
2 tablespoons walnuts, chopped

Procedure:

Get a bowl and combine all the ingredients, except the chopped walnuts. Adjust the taste before adding the chopped walnuts.

Vinaigrette: Rosemary and Orange

This recipe is also inspired by lemon vinaigrette.

Ingredients:

3 tablespoons fresh lime or lemon juice
Half teaspoon of Dijon mustard
3/4 cup olive oil, extra-virgin
1 orange, get the juice and grate the zest
1 teaspoon rosemary, chopped
Salt and ground black pepper to taste

Procedure:

Get a bowl and mix all the ingredients. Adjust the taste and infuse overnight.

Ginger Vinaigrette Asian Style

This vinaigrette is a good dressing for bitter greens or salads with roasted beets.

Ingredients:

1 large ginger, peeled and grated
3 tablespoons rice vinegar
2/3 cup olive oil, extra-virgin
1 tablespoons sesame oil
Salt and ground black pepper to taste

Procedure:

Squeeze the grated ginger to get 1 tablespoons of juice, discard the ginger after getting the juice. Combine the ginger juice and rice vinegar in a bowl. While whisking the ingredients in the bowl, add olive oil a little at a time. Put in the sesame oil and season to taste.

Classic Pan Seared Steak

It's impossible to go wrong with this pan seared steak. It is easy to prepare, succulent, and guilt-free. This is good for four persons.

Ingredients:

4 grass-fed rib eye steaks, about 10 ounces and 1-inch thick each
dry rub (combine: 2 teaspoons salt, 1 finely chopped onion, 2 teaspoons black pepper, 2 cloves minced garlic, 1 teaspoon paprika)
4 sprigs of rosemary
4 tablespoons clarified butter
1 whole garlic, peeled and minced
Coconut oil

Procedure:

1. Brush your room temperature steaks with some coconut oil to prevent the dry rub from escaping.

2. Coat each steak with the dry rub.

3. Set aside. Allow the meat to absorb the flavors of the dry rub.

4. Ready your cast iron pan and put it over high heat. When you see smoke, your pan is ready.

5. Put your steaks in the pan, and cook each side for 3 minutes for medium rare. You need to cook longer if you want it well done.

6. Set the cooked steaks aside, keep them warm by covering them with foil.

7. Put a pan over medium low heat, and add the steak drippings, butter, garlic cloves, and rosemary. Slightly brown the garlic, and

when the fragrance of rosemary fills the air you can turn off the heat and pour it over your steaks.

Serve your dish and enjoy.

Stir Fried Ground Beef with Cabbage

This recipe serves two to three people.

Ingredients:

2 pounds ground beef (preferably grass-fed)
1 cup water chestnuts, sliced
1 head Napa cabbage, julienned
3 cloves garlic, minced
1 clove garlic, minced
1/2 cup bamboo shoots, julienned
1 tablespoon fresh ginger root, julienne cut
3/4 cup coconut aminos
1/2 cup scallions thinly cut
2 tablespoons sesame seeds
Pinch of black pepper
2-3 tablespoons coconut oil

Procedure:

1. Get two pans – for the ground beef and the cabbage.

2. Put each pan on separate burners over medium heat.

3. Put 2 tablespoons oil in the ground beef pan and 1 tablespoon oil in the other pan.

4. You can now add the beef in the ground beef pan, and turn the beef occasionally as it cooks.

5. You can also add the cabbage in the other pan. Toss it until the oil covers the cabbage. Let it wilt.

6. Add the ginger over the half done beef, followed by bamboo shoots and water chestnuts.

7. Add 1 clove minced garlic on the other pan when you see that the volume has reduced. Coat the cabbage with garlic by tossing.

8. Add 3 cloves minced garlic in the beef pan. Slightly brown the beef.

9. Add 1/4 cup coconut aminos on the cabbage and reduce it a bit before serving.

10. In the ground beef pan, add in 1/2 cup coconut aminos, black pepper, and sesame seeds. Let the aminos reduce a bit.

11. You can remove either pan (or both pans) from heat after reducing the coconut aminos.

All-Time Favorite Meatballs

This recipe will yield around 18 meatballs.

Ingredients:

1 pound ground beef
4 pieces shiitake mushrooms, finely chopped
1/3 cup boiled sweet potatoes, mashed
1 tablespoon cilantro, finely chopped
1 small shallot, finely chopped
1 tablespoon tomato paste
Salt and pepper to taste
1 tablespoon coconut oil

Procedure:

1. Preheat the oven to 375°F.

2. Line your baking sheet with aluminum foil, and brush it with coconut oil.

3. Get a large bowl and toss the mushrooms, shallot, sweet potato, and cilantro in there.

4. You then add the ground beef, salt, pepper, and tomato paste.

5. Mix everything in the bowl well.

6. Form balls that measure 1 to 1 ½ inch in diameter.

7. Neatly arrange the finished meatballs on the baking sheet. Bake the meatballs for 10 to 15 minutes. You need to rotate the tray once in a while to ensure even cooking.

After baking, you can serve the meatballs or store them in your refrigerator after they have cooled.

Quick Pan Roasted Chicken

This recipe is quick and easy to prepare, and it is good for two people.

Ingredients:

3 large chicken thighs, halved
3 sprigs of thyme
A pinch of black pepper
1/2 teaspoon sea salt, finely ground
1/2 cup bone broth (whatever you have) with a splash of balsamic vinegar

Procedure:

1. Preheat the oven to 450°F.

2. Combine the sea salt and pepper – this will serve as your rub for your chicken thighs.

3. Get your oven-safe skillet, and put it over medium heat.

4. Sear the chicken pieces, skin touching the skillet, for three to five minutes.

5. When the chicken skin turned brown (not burnt), reverse the pieces and cook the other side for two minutes.

6. Add the broth and sprigs of thyme, and then put the skillet in the oven. Let the chicken roast for ten minutes or until tender.

Serve your dish and enjoy your meal.

Classic Chicken Liver Pâté

This recipe is easy to do, and you would want to savor it time and again.

Ingredients:

Half pound chicken livers
1 clove garlic, minced
3 slices of bacon, cubed
3 tablespoons sherry or vinegar
1 onion, diced
3/4 cup clarified butter
4 tablespoons parsley, chopped
Salt and pepper to season
Fresh nutmeg (optional)

Procedure:

1. Put the bacon on a large pan and cook over medium heat for three minutes.

2. Add in the garlic, onion, and 1/4 cup butter. Cook for another three to four minutes.

3. Prepare the chicken livers, remove the stringy part.

4. Put the livers to the pan and cook for 7 to 10 minutes. Add some more butter.

5. Add sherry, fresh nutmeg, parsley, salt, and pepper. Taste and adjust if needed.

6. Remove from heat and pour in a blender and blend until it reached a smooth consistency.

7. Pour the mixture in a dish.

8. Melt the remaining butter and evenly spread on the pâté.

9. Cover and keep in the refrigerator to cool, and to harden the fat.

You can also enjoy this pâté as a snack.

Paleo Coco-Vanilla Ice Cream

Yes, you can make a guilt-free ice cream to enjoy.

Ingredients:

1 can coconut milk, full-fat
4 egg yolks
4 tablespoons vanilla extract

Flavoring options:

your choice of berries, chopped or pureed
coconut flakes
chopped mint
chopped nuts
lemon, orange, or lime zest
raw honey
dark chocolate chips or flakes

Procedure:

1. Get a pot and boil some water, and then reduce the heat to simmer.

2. Create a double boiler by putting a heat proof bowl over it. Pour the coconut milk in the heat proof bowl. Add the vanilla extract, and heat it, but don't make it boil. If you choose to add mint or dark chocolate, it is the right time to add them now.

3. Get a separate bowl to whisk the egg yolks. Continue whisking the egg as you add the hot coconut milk by ladleful while keeping the eggs from being cooked in the hot coconut milk.

4. Pour the egg mixture into the double boiler, continue whisking.

5. Keep on whisking non-stop until you see a thick custard begins to form. Don't let it get too hot, and the simmering water must not touch the mixture.

6. When the custard is ready, you can now remove it from heat and let it cool on the table before you put it in the refrigerator.

7. You can add more flavoring later when the custard becomes cold enough to stick your finger in it.

8. Cool it more in the refrigerator, then put in the freezer.

9. Get your ice cream maker, follow its instructions, let your ice cream set. You can also try to put it in a baking dish, and take it out from the freezer to stir vigorously every 30 minutes. Do it for about 2 to 3 hours.

Enjoy your homemade guilt-free ice cream.

Quick Blueberry Dump Cake

This recipe is a must-try.

Ingredients:

1 pack Paleo-friendly yellow cake mix
1 teaspoon cinnamon, ground
1 cup coconut milk
Half cup ghee, melted
4 cups blueberries
Half cup coconut sugar

Procedure:

1. Preheat the oven to 350°F.

2. Get a baking dish and mix cinnamon, berries, and coconut sugar.

3. Get a bowl and put in the yellow cake mix and add coconut milk, mix them well.

4. Pour the yellow cake mixture over the berries, and pour ghee over the yellow cake mix without mixing.

6. Bake for 30 minutes or until slightly brown.

Let it cool before serving.

Fried Fish Curry

Ingredients:

2 pounds fillet of white fish
2 teaspoons curry powder
4 organic egg yolks
1/4 teaspoon pepper
1 teaspoon cumin
1 cup coconut, shredded
1 teaspoon salt
Lemon zest
Coconut oil

Procedure:

1. Make sure that your fish fillet is dry. Use a towel if you need to dry it.

2. Get a pan and put it over medium heat.

3. Add the coconut oil when the pan is hot enough, and make sure to cover the entire fish fillet.

4. As you wait for the cooking oil to get hot, get a bowl and whip the egg yolks.

5. Get a separate bowl, and add in the spices and coconut. Mix everything well.

6. Cover each fish fillet with egg, and then coat it with the coconut mixture.

7. Test if the oil is hot before deep frying the fish. Cook the fish until it turns golden brown.

Bacon, Mush, and Spinach

This dish is amazingly delicious that you might find it hard to believe that it's so simple to prepare.

Ingredients:

1 pound smoked bacon, cut into bite size strips
Half pound of button mushrooms, cut into four
2 cloves garlic, minced
2 handfuls of spinach, cut off the stems
1 onion, coarsely chopped
1 tablespoon lard
Dash of salt and pepper to taste

Procedure:

1. Get a casserole and put it over medium heat.

2. Add in the bacon, and let it release its natural fat. It is important not to make the bacon crispy.

3. Add the garlic, onion, and mushroom. Cook until the mushroom becomes tender.

4. Add spinach and lard.

7. Cover your casserole. Stir it occasionally, and cook until the spinach becomes tender.

8. Season it with salt and pepper. Serve.

Sweet Potato Fries Recipe

Ingredients:

2 pounds sweet potatoes, cut in wedges
1/4 cup coconut oil
2 to 3 teaspoons fresh or dried herb of your choice
Salt and pepper to season

Procedure:

1. Preheat the oven to 425°F.

2. Get a bowl and add in the oil and herbs. Add in the potato wedges and coat each piece with oil and herb mixture.

3. Add salt and pepper to season.

4. Align the wedges on a baking tray to cook evenly.

5. Cook the potato wedges for about 20 minutes.

6. Prick the wedges with the tip of your knife and see if they are tender enough to eat. If not, you need to cook them in the oven for another 5 minutes, and then test again.

Serve your sweet potato wedges and enjoy.

You can create simple soups with your frozen broth by adding your choice of vegetables and pre-cooked meat. You can also use the frozen broth for a tastier dish. You can mix and match the dishes in this chapter in planning your meal. You and your family will get to enjoy a healthy and great tasting meal all the time.

Chapter 5: Common Mistakes in Meal Planning for Crossfit Diet

Although Paleo diet is the most ideal diet program for a crossfitter to follow, you still need to modify it to meet the nutritional requirements of your body. Paleo could teach you how to eat clean and quality foods all the time. You can turn it into a habit in the long run.

Strictly Follows a Paleo Diet

If you are a crossfitter that does it for recreational purposes, then following a Paleo diet can give you a healthy and fit body without trouble. However, it is different if you are an athlete who intends to compete. If you are training rigidly for more than two hours a day, then your main source of energy is quality carbohydrates. The usual Paleo Diet does not provide enough carbohydrates to properly support your training. Even so, it does not mean you have to stuff your tummy with bread, sugar, and pasta just to get the carbohydrates that your body needs. Don't forget that you must consume quality carbohydrates (refer to the food guide list) as much as possible.

You can add "other" carbohydrates once in a while, but make sure that you have enough will power to stop yourself from craving too much bad carbohydrates. Sugar is definitely an enemy that you need to stay away from.

Finds it Hard to Believe that Diet Alone won't Do

Your diet plays a crucial role in providing your body with the right amount of nutrients it needs to support you during intense workouts. But, diet is not the only thing responsible for attaining success in your endeavor. Everything must be balanced. You need to have the right amount of exercise, the right foods, proper rest, healthy recreational activities, and other factors. You should not rely on your diet alone to give you the results that you want to see.

A Well Planned Diet Gives Faster Results

There are some people who spend so much time planning for the most ideal diet that could give them the results they want to see in just a few weeks. However, when they failed to see it most of them get frustrated and eventually stop doing the training and diet program all together.

Know that even if you have a well planned diet, you will not see a large impact within a few weeks. Your body is slowly changing from deep within, and you will not see it until after some months.

Create a well planned diet if you want, but don't expect to see immediate results. Don't stop doing what you have started just because you failed to see the expected results that you want to see within the time frame that you set. The moment you stop doing it, your body will only go back to the way it was before, and any initial improvement that already happened deep within will no longer manifest on the surface.

Plan a Meal that's Right for the Needs of your Body

When you plan your meal, make sure that you have enough of everything to give your body the nutrients it needs during the training. Don't create too much body fuel that you won't be able to burn, and don't deprive your body of the needed fuel when you have rigid workout. Eat the right amount of food with right proportion depending on the kind of training that you intend to do.

It might be a bit tricky to create the correct diet meal plan at first, but soon you will be able to discover the most efficient way of doing it. Also, don't forget to drink plenty of water to keep you hydrated.

Chapter 6: Sample Meal Plan

Below is a sample meal plan that you can try to get you started with your crossfit diet, you can modify it and add more carbohydrates if you train everyday for more than an hour:

	Breakfast	Lunch	Dinner	Snack
Mon	Berries and mixed nuts with coconut milk	Egg salad filled lettuce	Bacon, Mush, and Spinach	Macadamia nuts
Tues	Leftover Bacon, Mush, and Spinach	Chicken broth with veggies and liver pâté	Pan Seared Steak with roasted veggies	Beef jerky
Wed	Spinach omelet and onion with leftover liver pâté	Tuna salad in lettuce with almonds	Beef recipe with Coconut ice cream for dessert	Eggs (Hard boiled)
Thurs	Bacon and eggs with any kind of fruit	Beef recipe and Sweet Potato Wedges	Grilled trout and Paleo broth with some veggies	Smoked salmon
Fri	Smoothie (Coconut milk)	Stir Fried Ground Beef with Cabbage	Roasted chicken with fries (sweet potato)	Almonds and berries mix in a bowl
Sat	Roast chicken (Cold Leftover) with Paleo mayo	Meat balls and Coconut ice cream dessert	Fried Fish Curry and Blueberry Dump Cake	Can of salmon with olive oil & lemon juice
Sun	Stir-fry (Tomato and egg)	Fried pork chops with sautéed spinach	Chicken recipe	Olives & sauerkraut

Chapter 7: Hungry for more Information?

Here are some of the sites that can help you plan your meal, and other things that you need to know about crossfit.

For more recipes that you can include in your diet plan you can visit this site:

http://paleoleap.com/

If you want to know more about how to start a crossfit workout or training, then you can visit this site:

http://www.bodybuilding.com/fun/crossfit-q-a-your-guide-to-starting-crossfit.html

For your ingredients, it is best to visit stores that sell organic produce. Stay away from canned goods that contain chemical preservatives as much as possible. If you want to know more meal planning and the shopping list that you need to have, then you can visit this site:

http://crossfitlongbeach.com/meal-plan-shopping-list

You can have further reading if you go to this site:

http://theathleticbuild.com/diet-of-a-crossfit-athlete/

Start your crossfit diet now, and you will be glad that you did.

Conclusion

Thank you again for downloading this book!

I hope this book was able to help you to create the perfect crosfitter diet plan for yourself.

The next step is to continue practicing what you have learned from this book, and hopefully you will be able to influence your peers to do the same.

Finally, if you enjoyed this book, then I'd like to ask you for a favor, would you be kind enough to leave a review for this book on Amazon? It'd be greatly appreciated!

Click here to leave a review for this book on Amazon!

Thank you and good luck!